I0419735

Stop Emotional Eating!

An Introductory Guide to Ending

Emotional Eating Forever!

RON KNESS

Table of Contents

Introduction

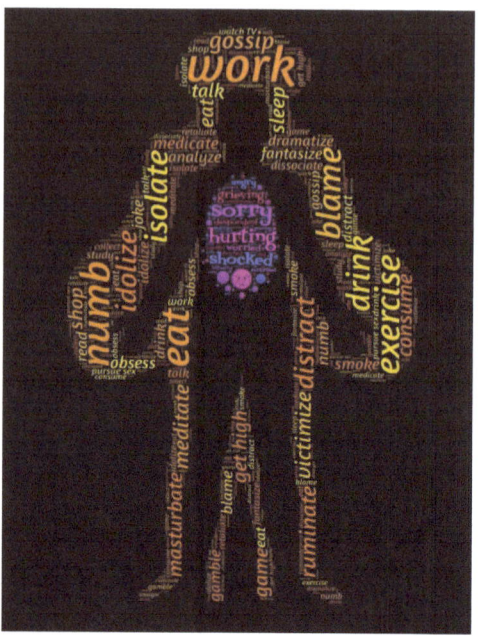

Do you find yourself gaining weight during times of stress? Do you fear boredom because you know you'll simply eat to fill the time? These are just some of the symptoms of emotional overeating and maybe the exact reason you have chosen to begin reading this guide.

Emotional overeating is almost a joke in our society - movies, TV shows, and the resulting stereotypes cause many of us to laugh about how much ice cream it takes to get over a boyfriend, or how much chocolate we need to overcome rejection. But for those who actually suffer from emotional overeating, it's anything but funny.

STOP EMOTIONAL EATING!

If you think you may suffer from this relatively common eating disorder, here are some signs and symptoms to begin with that may help you identify whether or not this is what you're struggling with.

Mindless Eating

If you have a binge eating disorder or emotional overeating problem, you may stuff food in and not even really taste it or realize what you're doing. It's as though you are "out of it" and just mindlessly stuffing food into your mouth.

Feelings of Guilt and Shame

Many people with emotional overeating disorders feel really embarrassed and hateful of themselves after they've got through with an eating binge. The problem, of course, is that these negative feelings may make you reach for more food for comfort. And the endless cycle continues ...

Eating in Secret

Because of being embarrassed, many emotional overeaters will eat in private, reserving their "naughty" foods for when no one is looking.

Always on My Mind...

Do you think about food all the time? Do you feel anxious about the prospect of leaving the house without snacks or money to buy food? Constantly thinking about food (food obsession) may be a sign that you have an emotional overeating disorder.

Feeling Sick

Sometimes, emotional overeaters will eat and eat to comfort themselves, and then feel sick afterward. Obviously, this is your body's way of telling you you've eaten far too much more than is good for you; but for emotional overeaters, this sickness does not necessarily deter the next binge.

Could Your Weight Gain Be the Result of Emotional Overeating?

Weight gain is frustrating enough, but when you can't seem to identify the cause(s) of it, because you're are eating and not even aware that you are doing it, the frustration is compounded. Emotional overeating is a somewhat sneaky problem - because it can involve mindless eating, it's the sort of thing that can occur without you realizing it. If you are having trouble figuring out what's causing your weight gain, here are some tips on identifying emotional overeating (as opposed to just overeating).

Seemingly Unexplainable Weight Gain

If you are gaining weight and you can't seem to figure out why, this is (ironically) a sign that the problem may lie with emotional overeating. As noted above, you often don't know you're doing it when it comes to emotional overeating. You may even be working out regularly and preparing healthy meals and still gaining weight, because you are mindlessly eating other foods when you feel negative emotions.

STOP EMOTIONAL EATING!

A Sudden Urge
Sources say that emotional "hunger" comes on quite suddenly, perhaps in the form of an irresistible craving for a certain food or just the urge to eat right now. True hunger is usually more gradual than that - unless you have low blood sugar or have gone a very long time without eating, true hunger does not usually take the form of an urgent need to eat a whole lot right away.

Depression
More and more the connection between emotional overeating and depression is being discovered. Do you feel depressed periodically? When you even think of feeling depressed, what goes through your mind? How do you cope? If you are picturing a big serving of your favorite comfort food, then this may be a sign that your overeating is emotion-based.

Stress
Are you going through a stressful time in your life simultaneous to your weight gain? Have you seen that pattern before? Stress, with its accompanying anxiety and other negative feelings, can trigger someone to overeat in response to those feelings.

Guilt
How do you feel after you eat? Are you consumed with guilt? Do you feel ashamed? These feelings are signs that you have a problem with emotional overeating. Normal eating to satisfy normal hunger does not make a person feel guilty.

Specific Cravings

As many parents know, genuine hunger usually means that you're more open to various food options. In emotional overeating, though, cravings may be so specific that no other food will do to satisfy your "hunger." You feel like you have to have that particular food to feel satisfied.

Do any of these signs and symptoms describe you and your situation? If so, don't despair – In this introductory guide to ending emotional eating we will be covering exactly how you can recognize the signs of emotional eating and how you can end it once and for all.

I hope you're excited, because I am…Let's get started!

Causes of Emotional Eating

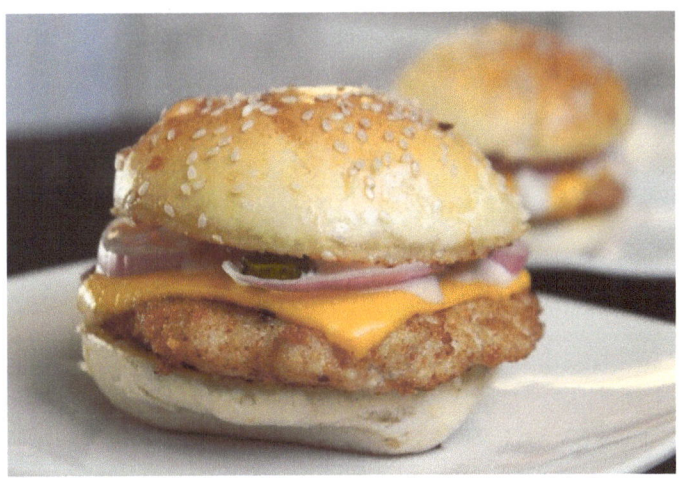

Emotional overeating disorders can be difficult and devastating for those who suffer from them. What makes this happen? Why is it that some people, knowingly or unknowingly, turn to food for comfort? Here are some thoughts and ideas on those questions.

At the core, emotional overeating disorder is a general term that refers to any of various eating habits where genuine hunger is not the motivational factor. It is more common among women than men, but men are not immune - especially young men in their teens and twenties. Those who suffer from this disorder associate food with emotional comfort, and will turn to eating to escape negative feelings.

Past Trauma

For some with emotional overeating disorder, the problem stems from past traumatic events. Someone who suffered sexual abuse, for example, or some other kind of sexual trauma may overeat in response to feelings of anxiety and confusion.

The result is a fatter body, which some sources suggest may cause the sufferer to feel "protected" from being attractive to the opposite sex. Subconsciously or consciously, the sufferer wants to be unattractive. Other examples of past trauma or unmet needs may cause a person to turn to emotional overeating.

Poor Self-Image

People who suffer from low self-esteem and a negative self-image may seek escape by overeating. In a way, emotional overeating is a physical expression of what the sufferer feels inside, and the resulting weight projects the same image of self-disrespect.

Self-Medication

Like alcoholics, those who struggle with emotional overeating may be unconsciously using food as a drug. Eating numbs or dulls the emotions that might be too hard to deal with otherwise.

Depression

As we have touched in in the introduction, Studies indicate a strong correlation between depression and emotional overeating. Ironically, sometimes as depression grows worse a sufferer loses weight; weight loss means the sufferer is not eating as much, and therefore not engaging in his or her coping mechanism.

Stress

Again, Prolonged, unrelieved stress can have a profound effect on the body. Stress stimulates the body to produce, among other chemicals, the hormone cortisol. Cortisol apparently has a hunger-stimulating effect, and as the stressful emotions increase along with the cortisol, a cycle of emotional eating can play out.

Identify Your Triggers

Emotional overeating is usually triggered by something - emotions, yes, but sometimes we need to be more specific than that. Identifying your personal triggers can go a long way toward helping you overcome the disorder that are not necessarily in the categories above. Some examples might be:

Emotional - Eating to relieve boredom, stress, or anxiety or as a way to overcome relationship problems. If any of these are your triggers, engage in other methods to relieve them other than eating. Anything that takes you mind off of eating.

It may take some experimentation to find what works for you.

Psychological - You may eat in response to negative, self-destructive thoughts. In this case, you'll have to work at not getting the negative thoughts in the first place. Professional help can help you find ways to turn negative thoughts into positive ones or at least non-self-destructive.

Environmental/Situational - You may eat simply because the opportunity is there. Also in this category is the habit of eating while doing another activity, such as reading or watching TV. Here again, awareness is the key. Recognize the event or action associated with your emotional eating. Either eliminate the event or action or find other ways to deal with it besides overeating.

Now that we have covered what exactly emotional eating is and how it can be causing stress, weight gain and a miserable life. The next part will be looking at how we can overcome this disorder and start living a stress free, healthy life. Let's get into it!

What You Eat Can Help Stop Emotional Eating

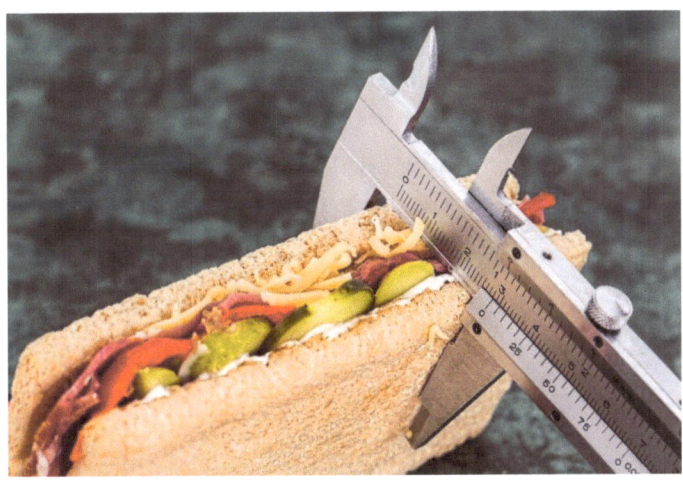

When you think of stopping emotional overeating, does it seem like an impossible goal? You're not alone - many people who suffer from this problem feel imprisoned and helpless. It can seem like you are unable to break free from the overwhelming emotions and habits. But there's good news, as we've just covered in the beginning of this guide.

Being honest with yourself is an important first step. Emotional overeaters tend to judge themselves pretty harshly, but don't - you're not an isolated case or some kind of freak. It's a sign of strength to seek help! It means you've identified the problem.

If you're struggling with this problem, there are some things you can do to get things under control.

1. Get advice from a therapist or specialist if you really want to find out if you are a victim of emotional overeating.

2. Keep a food diary. In this diary, in addition to noting everything you eat, also note how you feel when you eat - sad, angry, upset, elated, joyful, etc. Don't judge yourself or make any changes to your habits when you begin keeping this diary; you're not trying to impress anyone or prove anything. You are trying to get an honest picture of your eating habits. After several weeks, a pattern will probably emerge.

3. Your Grocery List - When an emotional moment hits and you head for the refrigerator or pantry, what kind of foods do you usually go for? Often, emotional overeaters head for high-calorie comfort foods like ice cream, chips, or candy bars. But you can't eat those things if they are not in your house!

Here are some examples of foods to put on your grocery list in place of the ones you may be tempted to buy. (Another tip - buy only the foods on your list. Compulsive buying of food is tempting.)

* Brown rice (instead of white rice)

* Millet (instead of or in addition to rice)

* Fresh fruits and vegetables (rather than canned)

* Low-fat, low-calorie yogurt (rather than ice cream)

STOP EMOTIONAL EATING!

* Popcorn kernels for air popping (rather than chips and fatty snacks)

* Lean protein like fish, turkey, and chicken (instead of deli meats and processed meats like hotdogs and bologna)

* Natural, healthy cooking oils like olive and safflower oil (instead of shortening, lard, or unhealthy oils)

Carrying on from the list above, Here is a short and quick list that can help ease out the grocery shopping process.

Protein

• Ham	• Turkey
• Veal	• Eggs
• Venison	• Buffalo Shrimp
• Lean Beef/Steak	• Swordfish
• Pork	• Salmon
• Lamb	• Tuna

• Chicken	• Cottage Cheese

• Meat: Beef, lamb, chicken and others. Grass-fed is best. These products are 100% real, unprocessed, and have a low-carb percentile.

You can cook these in coconut oil or you can even boil them and add them to your favorite vegetable soup. They are a great way to add lean protein to your diet. Just make sure you don't fry it or buy it with layers of fat. Ask for a lean cut piece when you go to the butcher.

• Fish: Salmon, trout, haddock, tuna and others. My personal favorites are the wild-caught fish. Again, they are unprocessed and have a very low percentage of carbs. Fish is recommended over meat simply because it has less fat. It has all the right nutrients and is 100% lean meat. You can make a tuna salad with some lemon, salt and pepper, or you can add it as a breakfast protein with a side salad or egg.

• Eggs: Omega-3 enriched or pastured eggs would be the best to eat. If you are looking for even better eggs, find a farm near you and buy from the farmer. It may cost a little more, but the results will be amazing. Again, protein is extremely important in a low-carb diet as you want to burn the fat and replace it with muscle to have a sexy lean figure. You can boil, fry (in coconut oil) or use it as an ingredient.

STOP EMOTIONAL EATING!

Carbohydrates/Vegetables/Fruits

• Celery	• Broccoli
• Parsley	• Cabbage
• Cucumber	• Spinach
• Peppers	• Asparagus
• Olives	• Peppers: green, yellow, red
• Romaine Lettuce	• Barley
• Onion	• Tomatoes
• Cucumber	• Oatmeal
• Yam	• Collard Greens
• Sweet Potato	• Carrots

• Apple	• Beans,
• Orange	• all types Brown Rice
• Squash	• Brussel Sprouts
• Quinoa	• Zucchini
• Cauliflower	• Lentils
• Green Beans	• Black eye Peas
• Garlic	• Legumes
• Artichokes	• Pineapple
• Yogurt	• Beets
• Avocado	• Peas

• Vegetables: Pretty much every vegetable known to man is low-carb and perfect for this lifestyle. You can make salads with spinach, kale, romaine lettuce, cauliflower, or even shredded carrots. Some have a higher glycemic index, therefore be careful with the portion sizes. They are full of vitamins though and can fill you up right away. Add some lean meats and proteins to your veggies for optimal results.

• Fruits: Fruits are tricky as they have natural sugar and therefore have a higher carb level. They are great for breakfast though; you can add them in your Greek yogurt, oatmeal, or just make a simple fruit salad. Again, careful with portion size.

Good Fats

• Udo's Choice Oil Blend	• Coconut Oil
• Flaxseed Oil	• Fatty Fish such as salmon, herring and trout
• Fish Oil Capsules	• Natural Peanut Butter
• Olive Oil	• Nuts and Seeds like Almonds

	Macadamia Oil

• Nuts and Seeds: Almonds, walnuts, sunflower seeds, etc. They are a great source of natural proteins and have a low carb percentage. You can add them to you fruit salads or to you vegetables and lean protein meal.

Fats and Oils: Coconut oil, olive oil, and cod fish liver oil. You might've stepped back a little with that last one, but they are all low-carb ingredients that can be added to your lean protein, salads, or cooking! They are full of nutrients that your body needs in order to function.

4. Don't Crash Diet

It's good to be proactive in solving problems, and emotional eating is no exception. If you try to crash diet, you may find yourself eating more after the crash diet is over. So, rather than stopping eating everything you love, try some of these tips.

* Allow yourself to have a dish of frozen yogurt each week as a treat. This approach tends to be easier than just cutting out all frozen treats.

You could use this approach with other "naughty" foods, too - it may be easier to resist if you know you are going to have that food on Saturday (or whatever day of the week you choose to have a small treat). The key is to control portion size!

* Boost your nutrition with a good quality vitamin and mineral supplement.

* Increase your consumption of nutrient-dense foods.

Eat Regular Meals

Experts recommend regular mealtimes as a way to combat emotional overeating. If it's not "time" for food, then you may be better able to hold off on eating until it is time. Also, eating regular meals helps you to be deliberate about your intake of nutritious foods.

And finally, having regular meal times tends to make for a more relaxed eating experience, which is the direct opposite of anxiety-driven overeating. In the next chapter we will take a look at the first step in overcoming emotional eating.

How Lifestyle Choices Affects Emotional Eating

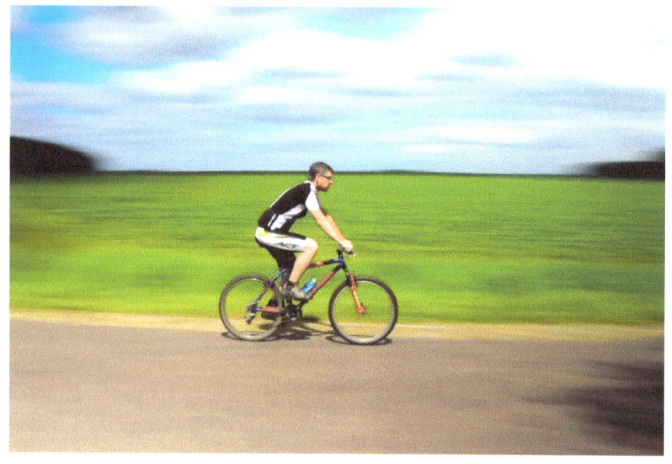

Overcoming emotional eating can seem overwhelming at the beginning, and setbacks can be expected. But the good news is, there are lifestyle choices that you can make to help overcome this problem.

The key word is choice - you can choose to follow a healthy lifestyle. Sometimes it helps to break things down into small, specific steps you can take (just trying to lead a "healthier lifestyle" is a bit vague!).

Following are some of these specifics. And remember, setbacks and relapses are not unusual.

Don't beat yourself up; you can't change what happened yesterday, but you can change what happens today and tomorrow. Just start fresh and drive on.

Exercise

Experts are in general agreement that regular exercise three to five days a week is most beneficial. This exercise should consist of at least 20 minutes of cardiovascular exercise (such as vigorous walking, jogging, biking, etc.) followed by some light toning or weight training.

Committing to this regimen full-force is not necessarily the best way to go; if you can only exercise once or twice a week, that's still better than nothing and will hopefully pave the way for more in the future.

Exercise is said to relieve emotional overeating in several ways. For one, exercise produces endorphins which are the body's natural "feel good" hormones.

For another, exercise prevents boredom and mindless eating, which is what you might be doing if you weren't exercising! And finally, exercise will likely boost your self-image, helping to break the cycle of low self-esteem and poor self-image that "feeds" emotional overeating disorder.

Nature

Never underestimate the healing power of nature! For those with emotional overeating disorder, choosing to spend more time out in nature can be particularly beneficial. After all, in the natural realm there are no media messages to mess with your self-image, and being in nature connects you to your origins and the origins of food.

Alternative stress relief

If you overeat in response to stress, it makes sense to find alternative ways to relieve and manage that stress. Meditation, Yoga, Pilates, martial arts, and other regular forms of exercise and relaxation techniques can help alleviate the stress that is triggering your overeating.

Swap goodies for goodies

Try to find substitutions for the comfort foods or food rewards you seek when you are feeling positive or negative emotions. Having something in place already is key - keep a list handy or other reminder that will prompt you to turn to the alternative rather than the candy bar. (Some alone time, a short walk, reading a magazine or book for pleasure, doing your nails, etc. are all little emotional pick-me-ups that you can implement in place of food.)

STOP EMOTIONAL EATING!

Why am I doing this?

Before eating, ask yourself why you are doing it.
Do you feel genuinely hungry? If you're truly hungry, you may feel fatigued and, of course, feel hunger in your stomach.

Ask yourself if you really feel hungry or if you are seeking an energy boost or a calming effect instead.

Lastly, some experts theorize that detachment from food and its natural source plays a role in emotional overeating disorder. Getting involved in nature and exploring and appreciating it can go a long way toward reconnecting with our biologically normal view of food.

Maybe you can kill two birds with one stone and do your regular exercise outdoors! Now that we have taken a look at lifestyle choices and how they can affect the way we eat, let's delve into different treatments to overcome emotional eating.

Is A Nutritional Deficiency Causing Your Emotional Eating?

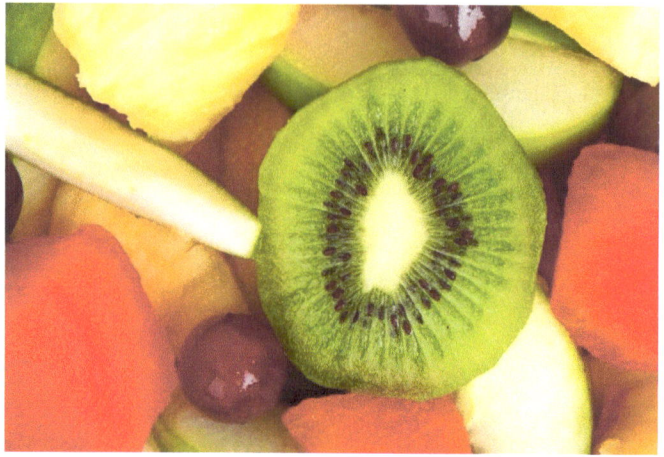

It may seem ironic to turn to nutritional treatments for emotional overeating - after all, isn't the problem too much eating? Why would you want to look at more foods you need to eat? But more and more experts are seeing the connection between nutrition and emotional overeating.

The fact is, when you overeat in response to emotions, you may not be eating the healthiest foods. You become full - even sick - on junk foods, and there's no room left for the good stuff. It's common knowledge that you do need the right nutrients to be healthy, and if those foods are not being eaten, then it's more a matter of quality than quantity.

Nutritional Deficiencies

Another aspect of emotional overeating may be nutritional deficiencies - and the deficiencies might bring on cravings. The theory is that the body craves certain foods in response to a need - in the case of emotional overeating, the need is emotional but it may also be physical. For example, a craving for ice cream may signify your body's need for calcium.

Here are some vitamins and minerals that, according to research, are implicated in the management of emotional overeating.

Vitamin D

This vitamin's effect on mood is well-documented, and is even suggested for people who suffer from certain depressive disorders, such as Seasonal Affective Disorder. Foods high in Vitamin D include:

* Cod liver oil

* Sockeye salmon

* Soymilk (fortified with Vitamin D)

* Cow's milk

Remember that Vitamin D is a fat-soluble vitamin, so sources with healthy fats, such as fish, may be absorbed better by the body. Or you can get a natural dose of Vitamin D by being out in the sun for 10 to 20 minutes, depending on your skin tone.

B-complex Vitamins

These important vitamins help increase energy levels and manage water retention. Foods with B vitamins include:

* Yogurt

* Eggs

* Lean beef (B12)

* Dark leafy greens (kale, broccoli, spinach)

Magnesium and Calcium

This is a powerful pair - many supplements put them together in one pill or capsule. These minerals are important for managing muscle and nerve tension.

Interestingly, when these minerals occur naturally in foods, there is usually a higher proportion of magnesium to calcium, whereas supplements generally have more calcium than magnesium. Foods include:

* Beans

* Nuts, especially peanuts, hazelnuts, and pecans

* Corn

Zinc

Zinc has been shown to have a profound effect on appetite and cravings, and many people with eating disorders are deficient in this mineral. Zinc is found in the following foods:

* Shellfish, especially oysters and crab

* Beef, particularly beef shanks

* Pork

* Chicken

* Garbanzo beans

Making deliberate, conscious choices about what you do eat can go a long way toward managing emotional overeating. Plan your meals and make a shopping list, and be proactive about meeting your nutritional needs.

Therapies That Can Help With Emotional Eating

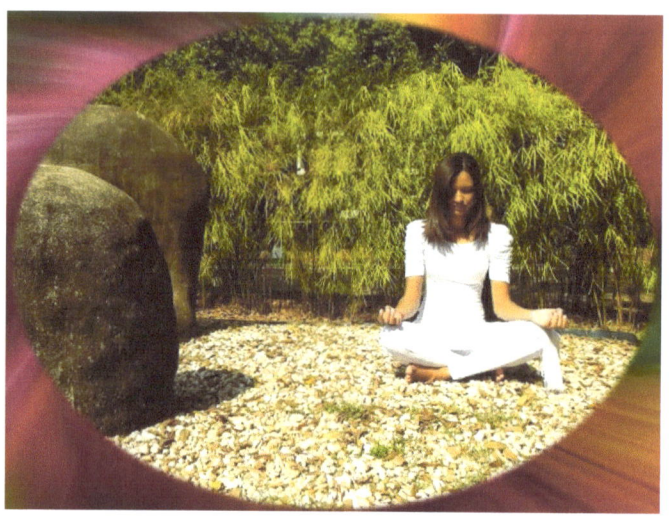

Emotional overeating can make a person feel imprisoned - it can seem like there is no way out of the cycle of feeling sad, angry, anxious and so forth, and then eating to alleviate the emotional pain.

There are treatments that are available, though - some of them conventional and some of them alternative.

Conventional therapy, surgery, and medication have all been utilized at one time or another for the treatment of emotional overeating. There are, however, some alternative therapies that are worth exploring. Here are some of them.

Hypnosis

Because emotional overeating begins in the mind, hypnosis is said to be effective because it addresses the mind directly with the power of suggestion. Hypnosis is not the mumbo-jumbo stuff of cartoons and swinging pocket watches; it's a clinical practice many practitioners have used with success to treat emotional overeating.

Meditation

The intent of meditation as a treatment for emotional overeating is to "tune in" to the emotional thought center that is driving your cravings and/or binge eating. Meditation, sometimes taking a form called "mindfulness," is the opposite of mindLESSness, which is what often happens in emotional overeating. The person does not really think about what he or she is doing; it's mindless eating.

Herbal Supplements

It seems like every time you turn around there's a new herbal supplement promising to help you lose weight. But there are some herbs that can help with the issue of emotional overeating. Here are some of them.

* Hoodia - This much-publicized herb is said to be effective at appetite suppression and boosting energy. Its effects tend to be subtle, and it also has a good safety record.

* Vitex - This hormone-balancing herb for women may help those whose emotional overeating is influenced by hormone fluctuations.

* Ginseng - This ancient herb is said to help sugar cravings and curb the compulsion to overeat in response to one's emotions. Both American and Asian ginseng are purported to be equally effective.

Acupuncture

Acupuncturists are often asked if acupuncture can help with weight loss. The answer, in general, is yes - but not always. However, the good news is that acupuncture tends to be more successful with treating emotional overeating than just overeating.

This may be due to acupuncture's alleged ability to release endorphins and boost metabolism - making the client feel better emotionally, effectively curtailing the emotional overeating.

Nutrition

As we've covered, having the right balance of vitamins and minerals may affect emotional overeating - it's not too much of a stretch to speculate that nutritional deficiencies could play a part in this kind of overeating. So make sure you're not eating a lot of artificial, processed, pre-packaged foods; opt for fresh, whole foods as a general rule.

It's also a good idea to take a vitamin and mineral supplement that is formulated for your gender and life situation. In the next chapter we will look at weight loss surgery and whether it is a viable option in overcoming emotional eating.

Weight Loss Surgery: Is It Right for You?

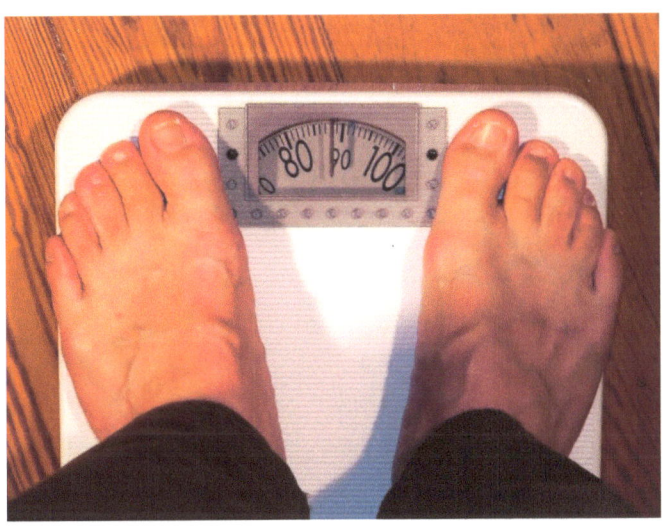

If you have trouble with emotional overeating, you may have considered weight loss surgery of some sort. But how do you know if it's for you? What kinds of surgery options are available?

Here are some ideas as to the more common surgical options currently available and some of the better-known pros and cons associated with them.

1. Lap-Band

This is a type of restrictive weight loss surgery, and it is adjustable. A silicon doughnut or ring is placed around the top of the stomach, leaving a small pouch above the ring. This is where the food goes first, and the pouch, being so small, fills up quickly. The person feels full on less food, in other words.

Slowly, the food makes its way from the pouch into the main stomach.

The doctor or surgeon may, from time to time, inject saline into the ring in order to inflate it, thus decreasing the pouch's capacity even further. The opposite can be done as well.

Pros:
* It's adjustable, as noted above - fluid can be removed or injected into the ring.
* The digestive process is not compromised; food is digested "the usual way."
* The surgical procedure is usually done laproscopically, meaning it's minimally invasive.

Cons:
* Additional surgery may be required in the case of twisting of the access port or perforation of the stomach.
* Weight loss tends to be rather slow and gradual, and not as dramatic as some other options.
* Repeated follow-up visits with your doctor are required.

2. Gastric Bypass
This is what's known as a malabsorptive technique. In gastric bypass surgery, a small pouch is created at the top of the stomach using "staples" rather than a ring. Then part of the small intestine is re-routed to connect to this pouch, essentially creating a permanently smaller stomach.

STOP EMOTIONAL EATING!

It is called "bypass" surgery because food bypasses the rest of the stomach and the original small intestine connection, called the duodenum.

Pros:
* Weight loss tends to be significant and permanent.
* Mild side effects, such as heartburn, tend to be resolved easily.

Cons:
* Compromised nutrient absorption is a significant concern, and patients are generally required to take many supplements to prevent nutritional deficiency.
* Dumping syndrome, or a too-fast emptying of stomach contents, is a potentially difficult side effect.
* It's harder for doctors to view the stomach and intestine via endoscopy, meaning cancer and other problems may go undetected.

These are just two of the more common types of weight loss surgery. The bottom line is, weight loss surgery can help with the weight gain and excessive caloric intake associated with emotional overeating, but it does not address the underlying emotional issues.

If you do choose some sort of surgery to treat emotional overeating, it's a good idea to make sure it's part of a "whole person" treatment plan that includes counseling and emotional therapy.

In the End ...

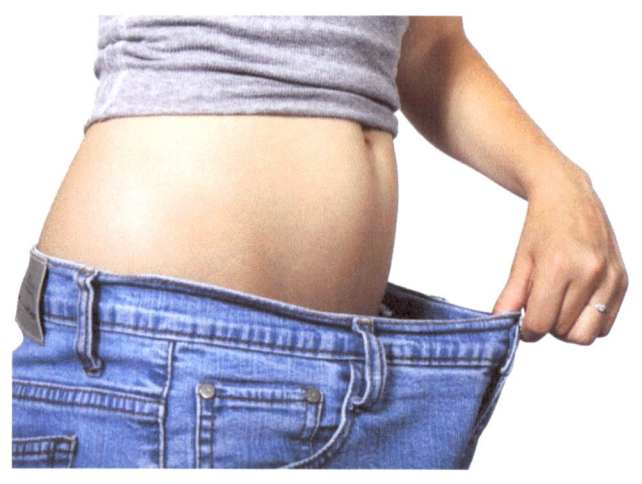

Well, we've made it to the end of our introductory guide to overcoming emotional eating and clarified why you may be overeating and gaining weight without knowing why. Hope you've enjoyed it!

In conclusion, emotional overeating can seem like a prison with no way out, and when you do think of seeking treatment, it can seem too overwhelming to consider. Sometimes it helps to have some simple steps and treatment programs laid out clearly, so it doesn't seem so overwhelming.

Following is a summary list of common treatment options for emotional overeating disorder, as well as some tips on things you can do and some cautions on what not to do.

Common Treatments

First, recognize your problem. Know you're not alone - the number of people who suffer from emotional overeating disorder is significant.

* **Counseling** - Individual, group, or family counseling can prove very helpful for people who experience emotional overeating. Counseling treatment usually involves some nutritional and dietary guidelines and treatment of underlying emotional problems.

* **Surgery** - This is a somewhat controversial treatment for emotional overeating - it addresses the physical aspect of the problem rather than the emotional. However, in combination with emotional therapy and extensive medical counseling, surgery is a viable choice for some sufferers. Usually, surgical options involve decreasing the space available in the stomach, usually by a lap-band or gastric bypass procedure.

* **Medication** - Under the care of a professional, medications - usually anti-depressants - have been shown to provide relief for many who suffer from emotional overeating. This may be due to the suspected connection between overeating and depression - research continues to point to the relationship between the two problems.

Extra Tips - What You Can Do

* **Exercise regularly** - Yes, you've heard this one, but it's really an important aspect of managing emotional overeating.

Exercise may improve mood, improve energy levels, and increase your self-image - all part of overcoming emotional overeating. You can start with just 20 minutes of brisk walking three to six times a week.

* **Eat well** - What you do eat is as important as what you're "not allowed" to eat! Sometimes, emotional overeaters can be overcome by cravings for certain "forbidden" foods, like ice cream, candy bars, and potato chips.

But if you're full of and surrounded by healthy foods, you can dig in without feeling guilty. Keep fresh produce on hand and eat lots of lean protein, veggies, fruits, and whole grains.

What Not to Do

* **Keep unhealthy snacks handy** - If you don't have the unhealthy food in the house, you will probably be less likely to head for it in times of emotional distress. In other words, make it hard on yourself to get the foods you want to eat when feeling bad - cross ice cream, junk foods, and fatty snacks off your grocery list.

* **Crash diet** - Trying to starve yourself or go on an extended fast is not recommended. You may compromise yourself nutritionally and/or physically, and crash dieting tends to result in more overeating afterward.

Well I hope our introductory guide has given you a great overview of emotional eating and steps to overcome it. If you believe you do have a problem that needs further attention please seek help from a trusted therapist or counsellor. Good luck for the journey and begin today!

About the Author

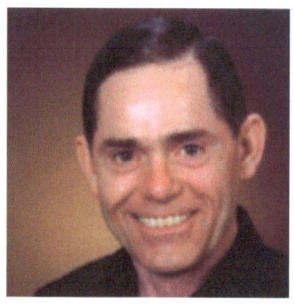

I grew up in Central Minnesota, where my parents own and operated a fishing resort. Once out of high school I tried a couple of semesters of college, only to quit halfway through the Spring term; I decided at that time that college wasn't for me.

Then I decided to follow my father's previous occupation as an auto mechanic. I graduated from a two-year of vocational training course and worked as a mechanic. While in vocational training, I decided to join the National Guard where I eventually ended up working full-time for 32 years.

So how does all of this relate to writing? In one of my leadership schools, the instructor, who was an English teacher at a juvenile detention center, presented writing to me in a whole new way - a way that started to develop my interest in working with words.

Fast forward about 40 years and I now have over 20 books listed on Amazon for Kindle. All of my books with the exception of one children's book (One, Two,

STOP EMOTIONAL EATING!

Three, Four . . . Counting is Fun at the Grocery Store) are non-fiction in various fields, such as:

*Health and Fitness:

- What You Eat Can Hurt You

- Eat Healthy to Lose Weight

- The Extreme Weight Loss Plan

- Get Ripped Abs

- Walking Down the Road to Fitness

- Design Your Ultimate Fitness Program - Walking

- A Healthier You in the Coming Year

- Senior Fitness – A Guide to Staying Young Beyond Your Years

- Managing Type 2 Diabetes Using Alternative And Natural Therapies

- How Diet and Exercise Can Better Manage Type 2 Diabetes

- The Low Carb Diet: A Beginner's Guide to Weight Loss Through Carbohydrate Management

- Arthritis – Live With Less Pain and Inflammation

* Self-Publishing:
- Writing for the Kindle

- How to Self-Publish Your Ebook on Amazon

- Pillars of Gold

- Kindle Advanced Strategies

- Self-publishing - Work Smarter, Not Harder

- The Home-Based Entrepreneur's Guide to Blogging

* Digital Photography:
- The Digital Photography Interactive Quiz

- How to Improve your Travel Photography

- Digital Photography: Aperture, Shutter Speed and You

- Don't Be In the Dark About Light

- The No Nonsense Guide to Digital Photography

- The Beginner's Guide to Digital Photography

- Digital Photography – A Quick Guide to Using Adobe Photoshop Elements

- Improve Your Blog Posts With Photos

- Digital Photography Anthology

STOP EMOTIONAL EATING!

* Travel:
- Travel Advisor

- Travel Trips and Tips

*Outdoors and Recreation:

- Making Your First Fly Rod

- The Beginner's Guide to Fly Tying

- Hooked on Fly Fishing

- The Secrets to Fly Fishing for Trout

- Tent Camping – The Ultimate in Family Fun

- Maintaining a Salt Water Pool

* Misc.:
- Making Wine from Kits

- Create Your Home Inventory

- The 9 Secrets to Using Your GI Bill Benefits

- The Life and Times of the Honey Bee

- The Military Spouses Financial Guide to Funding Education

- The Home-Based Entrepreneur's Guide to Blogging

- Survival Basics – Are You Prepared to Survive?

Besides my own writing, I also ghostwrite ebooks, reports, articles, blogs and do Kindle conversions for my clients.

Oh . . . did I mention that I went back to college in 1987 and graduated 7 years later?

Today my wife and I live in Gold Canyon, AZ, where you'll find me happily sitting in my office typing away on my laptop as I work on my next book or ghostwriting project . . . that is if we are not traveling on a cruise ship - our new-found mode of travel.

If you like my books, please leave a review of them on Amazon at the book links where purchased.

STOP EMOTIONAL EATING!